ALSO BY BERNIE KEATING

When America Does It Right

Riding the Fence Lines

Buffalo Gap Frontier

1960's Decade of Dissent: The Way We Were

Songs and Recipes: For Macho Men Only

Rational Market Economics

Music: Then and Now

A Romp thru Science

Riding My Horse

Searching for God

Chasing Tumbleweeds

Ebenezer Sackett's Christmas Carol

They Rode with Custer

Echoes

Pivot to Asia

My AUTOIMMUNE STUFF

BERNIE KEATING

authorHOUSE

AuthorHouse™
1663 Liberty Drive
Bloomington, IN 47403
www.authorhouse.com
Phone: 1 (800) 839-8640

Published by AuthorHouse 10/14/2017

ISBN: 978-1-5462-1226-3 (sc)
ISBN: 978-1-5462-1224-9 (hc)
ISBN: 978-1-5462-1225-6 (e)

Contents

PREAMBLE

Most of us spend our lives with little thought about death, other than religious things like: "going to heaven."

Suddenly, you find you have a serious disease; reality comes fast. What are the effects of the disease, to whom do you turn, what is the prognosis? You are shocked and emotions are overwhelming.

I have gone through that panic three times: seven years ago with an erroneous diagnosis of multiple myeloma later withdrawn, then with a diagnosis of dermatomyositis, and recently with a confirmed diagnosis of multiple myeloma; hence, I am now inflicted with two horrific autoimmune diseases. The final one was a shock, but this time I am better prepared to handle the emotions because "I know the territory" and have a reasonable strategy for treatment.

How do you become educated about your disease? The intent of this book is to be of assistance to someone like me who is undergoing a medical shock and seeks information and assurance.

Don't fail to read the final climatic chapter when I found I had the grave-maker: multiple myeloma. My end game is eight months, forty-eight, or "whatever"; it remains to be determined.

Bernie Keating

1

PANIC

It all began on the phone with my doctor. Then I called to my wife.

"Aurdery, the doctor said I may have multiple myeloma. It couldn't be worse. The disease is horrific with less than a year to live. We have to talk."

"Oh Bernie! My God. Oh! Oh! Dear God, what can we do?"

That was seven years ago and began discussions about how to handle life as an invalid, how to react to my death, and how to tell our children; there were no good answers - we ended with a prayer.

At eighty, I had never encountered a previous medical crisis.

Symptoms developed slowly. When a rash on my backside appeared, I went to Prompt Care where a doctor prescribed a dose of Prednisone and told me to see my family doctor. Of course I did not do that – who does? The rash was already gone and a-thing-of-the-past. The rash reoccurred two months later when I was visiting my daughter in Virginia; I went to their Prompt Care and they gave me the standard dose of Prednisone and told me to see my family doctor. Then a month later back home in Sonora it reoccurred for the third time and I finally went for an office visit with my family doctor, Lynn Austin MD.

After hearing the scenario of my reoccurring rashes, he offered the opinion that I have some sort of systemic problem and started me on a series of tests for various diseases including diabetes, hepatitis, tests to determine which kind of hepatitis, rheumatoid arthritis, lupus, and finally a test that indicated a possible diagnosis of multiple myeloma.

Three days later in midmorning I received a phone call at home from Doctor Austin.

"Good news, Bernie. I sent the test results to a local pathologist and just got the results back. He told me he could not find the particular things that would indicate multiple myeloma; so, I guess you dodged that bullet." He paused while I caught my breath.

"Now we will start some further tests to find out what systemic disease you have. You do have something. I will conduct certain tests they can't analyze here at the local lab that we send back to the Mayo Clinic, so it may take time before we get the results. If you will drop over to the blood draw tomorrow morning, we will get the process started."

My strength was deteriorating rapidly; I used a cane to walk and felt ill and weak. Only motivation kept me out of a wheel chair. When I went to the emergency ward they immediately put me in the hospital.

A day later, Doctor Austin entered my hospital room.

"Good news, Bernie, I have the results and a diagnosis. It is an autoimmune disease with the name Dermatomyositis. The CK test results should be below 300 and your result is 1230 - way above any normal range. It is an illness in which the white blood cells that are supposed to fight infections instead attack the skin and the muscles of your body; so, that is why you are getting rashes plus the muscle problems that have put you in the hospital. It is a rare disease; in my practice, I have seen only one other case."

I did not know how to react – was this diagnosis good or bad?

"I will contact Stanford Hospital in Palo Alto who have a special team for these autoimmune diseases and see if they will accept a referral from me. I think they may, because that is where I did my residency. I might have enough clout to get them to accept my referral."

Those rashes started in March, 2010, eight years ago and were the first symptoms of the medical ordeal that continues to this day.

There is no more dramatic emotional experience than finding you have a serious disease. What is the disease and what does this mean? It was the first time in my long life I ever faced this reality. My wife stood at my side and suffered all the same emotions.

The family doctor is the only lifeline available and became the center of my attention. How many life and death decisions like this for other patients had he gone through before; how many others had he saved - or ushered into death?

Dr. Lynn Austin was a unique guy and I was fortunate to have him as my primary physician. A graduate of the Mayo Clinic Medical School, he received a PhD in Physical Biochemistry at the University of California, Berkeley (I am an alum of their graduate school), and then did his residency at the Stanford Medical Hospital in Palo Alto.

He lived an unorthodox out-of-the-box life for a physician. True to his Mid-western roots he was a motorcyclist and took pride in riding his cycle to the annual Sturgis Rally. He was a gentleman rancher and operated a small cattle ranch outside Sonora. One morning during my office appointment he told me he had already delivered a calf on his ranch earlier that morning.

Hanging on his office wall was a certificate of membership in Sigma Xi, and it happened that both he and I had been voted membership in the Berkeley Chapter of Sigma Xi, a prestigious scientific honorary with membership that included a half-dozen Nobel Laurates, including Glenn Seaborg.

I went to Berkeley graduate school during the 1950's era of the "silent generation", and Lynn Austin a decade later in the 1960's era of hippies and Vietnam War. After he saw the front cover of my novel, *1960's Decade of Dissent*, which had the picture of a beautiful girl in hippy attire with headband, he said: "Bernie, I think I dated that girl".

Several years ago when he was 67 with 38 years of doctoring, he opted for other pastures and decided to retire. I was saddened to see him go and hope he has found a life in retirement that he richly deserves – I owe him much.

2

DERMATOYMYOSITIS

Let's look at my new illness. Dermatomyositis is an autoimmune disease that occurs when a body's immune response turns against healthy cells. It is an inflammatory disorder that weakens muscles and creates a painful skin rash over much of the body. Symptoms may occur suddenly or develop slowly over several months and often includes weight loss, fever, and lung inflammation.

It is an autoimmune disease with the cause unknown. There is no cure. Diagnosis is typically based on some combination of symptoms, blood tests, and muscle biopsies. The only known treatments involve various kinds of medications. Corticosteroids, principally prednisone, are typically used in an initial treatment and other agents like methotrexate or azathioprine are utilized if steroids are not working well. IVIG infusions of Intravenous immunoglobulin are sometimes employed and may improve outcomes. [1]

This autoimmune condition usually first occurs with those in

---

[1] "Dermatomyositis", Wikipedia, 2017

5

their 40s and 50s and women are affected more often than men; however, people of either sex or age may be affected. [2] The onset of my own disease at the elderly age of 80 is unusual.

It is a rare disease that is characterized by inflammation of the muscles and the skin. The immune system normally attacks foreign invaders, but instead with this disease it attacks the body's own skin and muscles. My initial encounter was a rash along my back, which was treated in Prompt Care with a six-day regimen of the steroid, prednisone. The rash extended all across my back with considerable itching. Prednisone provided temporary relief from the itching and the rash initially faded. This was followed a couple weeks later with a second and third reoccurrence and I again used treatment with prednisone. My legs became so weak that I resorted to the use of a cane for support and to maintain stability. I was on the verge of climbing into a wheel chair.

Realizing I was quite ill, I went to the emergency ward at the local hospital and I was immediately placed in a hospital bed and admitted as a patient. In the hospital I was medicated with a large dose (80 mg.) of prednisone that brought temporary relief but did little to treat the underlying disease.

With the assistance of Dr. Austin, my local Sonora internist, I was able to obtain a referral to a Stanford Health Care Clinic team in Redwood City that dealt with auto-immune diseases. My first appointment with the Stanford team was on October 20, 2010. Dr.

---

[2] ibid

David Fiorentino, dermatologist, was the principle examiner and practitioner at the Stanford Health Care clinic and he was joined by Dr. Lorinda Chung, immunologist. My first office visit at the clinic was a new and unnerving experience for me. Fortunately, I was accompanied by my wife, Aurdery, who took notes because I was overwhelmed to remember much of what transpired.

During an initial office visit, a patient learns little about their disease because of so many other distractions. The doctor's focus is on the diagnosis, assessing the patient's condition, and developing and outlining a treatment plan. The doctor has little time to spend educating the patient on the nuances of the disease. So it is up to the patient to find an effective means to educate him or her. Many people have no interest, or the ability, in learning details about their disease and they rely solely on a sketchy understanding; however, I feel the more you learn about the cause and symptoms, the better you will be able to respond to treatment. Let me provide what I have learned about my disease after accomplishing research on the internet, coupled with seven years of actual experience. [3]

At the outset I should admit to a lack of understanding of organic chemistry, which is much more complex than the inorganic chemistry I studied in college seventy years ago; hence, beware of my descriptions, but a vague understanding of organic chemistry may be better than none at all: it is a crucial element of my disease.

The exact cause of dermatomyositis isn't known. This

---

[3] ibid

autoimmune disease occurs when your body's disease-fighting cells, called antibodies, attack your healthy cells. Having a corrupted or altered immune system may contribute; for example, having a viral infection or cancer may damage your immune system and lead to development of the disease.

The most important component of the immune system is the marrow inside the bone. It is an important chemical factory of the body where both red and white blood cells are produced. The bone marrow is a busy place where many proteins live. These proteins are large organic molecules composed of long chains of amino acids (sub-components of proteins) and are often linked end-to-end. These proteins in the bone marrow perform an array of critical functions within the human body. Their functions differ from one another and are controlled by the genes in a person's chromosome. It is their normal job to manufacture two types of antibodies (immunoglobulin): red blood cells and white blood cells.

Some of these proteins produce red blood cells that pass through the passageways of the bone wall to enter the blood stream and carry the oxygen picked up and supplied by the lungs to all of the muscles and tissues throughout the body. These red blood cells provide this vital oxygen to all the organs throughout the body including the brain, all the muscles, and other body tissues.

The other proteins in the bone marrow produce a type of white blood cell (called plasma cells) whose normal function is to enter the blood stream in a defensive action whenever a foreign invader attacks the body. It is these white blood cells that have become corrupted or altered by the disease. Unfortunately, these corrupted white blood cells begin to attack the skin and muscles instead of fighting foreign invaders, such as infections.

What caused the proteins in the marrow that produce white blood cells to become altered is unknown. Perhaps a viral infection or cancer is the cause. It is not uncommon to find a cancer of some kind that exists somewhere in the body; so, that may be an underlying cause. During my initial medical going-over, I received extensive tests looking for cancer throughout my entire body to determine if that was a cause. I was given a colonoscopy examination, CAT scans, endocrine ultra sound of the pancreas through the stomach wall, and other tests. After these exhaustive tests, no cancer was found anywhere in my body, so that was ruled out as a cause.

The corrupted white blood cells cause skin rashes and weakened muscles. These include not only the external arm and leg muscles but also the many other internal muscles throughout the body that performs functions such as swallowing and control over the small intestines, colon, and rectum. We tend to take these internal reflexive muscles almost for granted, but I quickly found that was a mistake since they have major impact on my own human activities.

In most cases with the onset of the disease, the first symptom is a distinctive skin rash on the face, chest, nails, or elbows. The rash is patchy and usually a bluish-purple color. This occurred three times during the initial stages of my disease, each time separated by a month with intervening visits to Prompt Care where I obtained temporary relief with the use of the steroid, prednisone.

I also had muscle weakness that grew worse over time. This weakness started in my neck, arms, and hips and was experienced on both sides of my body. In addition to weakness, I felt so ill that I went to the local hospital emergency ward and was immediately placed in a hospital bed and admitted for treatment. Some of the symptoms I experienced were:

Muscle pain.

Muscle tenderness.

Problems swallowing.

Lung problems.

Hard calcium deposits underneath the skin.

Fatigue.

Unintentional weight loss.

Fever.

Control of unpredictable bowel movements became a major issue for me. As a result of the loss of muscle control of my colon and rectum, I was unable to have power over or even predict the activity of bowel movements. I received little advance indication (sometimes less than three seconds) that a bowel movement was about to occur. This created considerable hygiene and social problems and made me virtually a captive of a nearby bathroom. I immediately retired my normal under-garments and opted for the throwaway type. The problems associated with digestive health will be discussed in a later chapter.

There's no cure for dermatomyositis. A remission is possible, but this is rare. Effective treatment with medications can improve the condition of your skin and muscles and it is possible to maintain a satisfactory quality-of-life.

Medications perform a vital and almost the only significant role in treating dermatomyositis. It is with use of medications that a person can survive and even obtain a reasonably satisfactory quality-of-life. There is virtually no other means of treatment than through the use of various medications and infusions. The use of medication will be discussed in a later chapter.

3

IMMUNE SYSTEM

Until I encountered immune problems, I knew practically nothing about the complex immune system, and confess it is still somewhat of a mystery to me. It is a difficult area for medical science to study because of its biochemical complexity and many of its functions occur in the exotic chemical factory of the marrow. This marrow inside bones is the primary component of the immune system.

Even though the immune system is exceeding complex and beyond my biochemical expertise to fully understand, permit me to describe the normal way it is supposed to operate as I have researched and attempted to understand it from information in various websites. [4]

The starting place for understanding the immune system is the marrow inside bones. The makeup of this marrow consists of proteins, which are large bio-molecules (polypeptides) that consist of one or more long chains of amino acids (the chief sub-structures

---

[4] "immune System:, Wikipedia 2017

of proteins). [5] Proteins consist of one or more polypeptides arranged in a biologically functional way. These proteins perform an array of functions within organisms. They differ from one another, which is dictated the genome; hence, like so many other functions within the human body, it is the genes that ultimately determine the structure and activity of these proteins.

Within the bone marrow, amino acids form large protein molecules called a polypeptide. A polypeptide is a long, continuous molecular chain, often linked end-to-end, consisting of amino acids. These protein molecules chemically will produce red blood cells (hemoglobin) that carry oxygen picked up in the lungs to the muscles throughout the body, and other proteins produce white blood cells (plasma cells) that fight infections. [6]

Red blood cells are the most common type of blood cell and the principal means of delivering oxygen to the body tissues by the blood flowing through the circulatory system. These red blood cells take up oxygen in the lungs and release it into tissues while squeezing through the body's capillaries. They are rich in hemoglobin, an iron-containing biomolecule that can bind oxygen and is responsible for the red color of the cells. They provide properties essential for physiological cell functions that support life. These red blood cells develop in the bone marrow and circulate for about 120 days in the body before their components

[5] "Peptides", Wikipedia, 2017

[6] ibid

are recycled. Approximately a quarter of the cells in the human body are red blood cells. [7]

White blood cells (also called leukocytes) are the cells of the immune system that are involved in protecting the body against both infectious disease and foreign invaders. All white blood cells are produced and derived from cells in the bone marrow known as (hematopoietic) stem cells. Leukocytes are found throughout the body, including the blood and lymphatic system. [8]

The immune system is the defense system within the body that protects against disease. An immune system must detect a variety of pathogens (viruses or bacterium) and distinguish them from the organism's own healthy tissue. [9]

Lymphatic System:

The lymphatic system is part of the circulatory system and a vital part of the immune system, comprising a network of vessels that carry a clear fluid called lymph. The lymphatic system, unlike the circulatory system, is not a closed system and one of its functions is to provide a return route for the blood in the circulatory system.

The other main function of the lymphatic system is defense in the immune system. Lymph is very similar to blood plasma; it contains lymphocytes and other white blood cells. It also contains

---

[7] "Red Blood Cells", Wikipedia 2017

[8] "White Blood Cells", Wikipedia 2017

[9] "Immune System", Wikipedia, 2017

waste products and cellular debris together with bacteria and proteins. Lymphocytes are concentrated in the lymph nodes. [10]

The lymphatic system is a component of the immune system. If I ever encountered it during high school biology, I guess I forgot almost everything I had learned. It is a key extension of the immune system with its principle components outside the bone, comprising a network of lymphatic vessels that carry a clear fluid called lymph. This is a fluid very similar to blood plasma; it contains lymphocytes (plasma cells that initiate the immune response). It also contains waste products and cellular debris of bacteria and proteins for discharge from the body. [11]

These constituents of lymph fluid and blood from the marrow exit the bone through the Microvascular Exchange Blood Vessels ("vascular" passageways through the wall of the bone). I had previously thought the wall of the bone was impregnatable, but now realize the blood and lymph flow through the wall of the bone utilizing these passageways.

Lymph is a fluid formed in the marrow, passes through the vascular passageway, and enters the vessels of the lymphatic system. Eventually, the lymph vessels empty into the lymphatic ducts, which include lymph nodes.

Lymph nodes are located along the lymphatic system. There are hundreds of lymph nodes grouped in clusters in different regions

---

[10] "Lymphatic system", Wikipedia, 2017

[11] ibid

(groin, armpit, neck). A lymph follicle expands significantly when encountering a foreign antigen, which is why a doctor checks for swollen lymph nodes when you report an illness. A swollen lymph node suggests some sort of infection.

Pathogens (infections) can rapidly evolve and adapt and thereby avoid detection and neutralization by the immune system; however, multiple defense mechanisms have also evolved to recognize and neutralize pathogens. Acquired immunity creates memory after an initial response to a specific pathogen, leading to an enhanced response in subsequent encounters with that same pathogen. This process of acquired immunity is the basis of vaccination. [12]

Disorders of the Immune System:

Disorders of the immune system can result in *autoimmune* diseases, inflammatory diseases, and cancer. *Immuno-deficiency* occurs when the immune system is less active than normal resulting in recurring and life-threatening infections. It can either be the result of a genetic disease or acquired conditions such as HIV/AIDS. In contrast, *autoimmunity* results from a hyperactive immune system attacking normal tissues as if they were foreign organisms. Common *autoimmune* diseases include dermatomyositis (attacks skin and muscles), rheumatoid arthritis

---

[12] "Immune System", Wikipedia, 2017

(attacks joints), diabetes mellitus type 1(insufficient insulin), and systemic lupus (attacks various internal organs). [13]

There, does that explain the immune system? I told you it was complex and only partially understood by me.

---

[13] ibid

4

STANFORD HOSPITAL

Having received my Master Degree in graduate school at the University of California, Berkeley, it was intimidating for me to place myself at the mercy of archrival Stanford University and their hospital for my medical care; however, my grandson had been successfully treated at their Lucile Packard Children's Hospital for Leukemia. The Stanford Hospital had a sterling reputation. I was fortunate when they accepted a referral from Doctor Austin for my treatment. (He did his residency there.)

My initial encounter was at their Stanford out-patient clinic in Redwood City with a team of specialist for autoimmune diseases that included Doctor David Fiorentino, a Dermatologist, and Doctor Lorinda Chung, an immunologist. In addition to proving leadership to the team in the clinic, they are actively involved in guiding research programs, and both are Professors who teach at the Stanford School of Medicine. This inter-discipline team was able to bring to bear the latest expertise and research relative to immune diseases.

My first appointment was on October 20, 2010 with Dr. David Fiorentino. It was a new and unnerving experience for me. Fortunately, I was accompanied by Aurdery who took notes because I was overwhelmed to remember much of what transpired.

Stanford is a teaching hospital in which new doctors in residency are educated hands-on in the medical field. Prior to an examination of a patient by the full team, a doctor in residency conducts a preliminary exam of the patient. The specialist team then listens to the details found by the resident in private, and then the team conducts their own thorough exam to confirm the findings. Doctor Fiorentino was the principle examiner. The following was the procedure as I remember it.

1. Inasmuch as the disease involved both the skin and muscles, the initial examination was to assess the status of both. The skin of my body, head to toe, was carefully examined, which included the location and appearance of all areas of rash or other skin conditions.

2. I was given physical strength tests for all my muscles, including arms, wrists, legs, ankles, and feet. This included lying on my back on the examining table, rolling over onto my stomach and additional strength tests. Each muscle was given a rating of 0 to 10. I had previously been spending an hour/day in aerobic exercise at the Sonora Fitness Gym, so my muscles were in good physical condition and most of my ratings were a 9 or 10.

3. Doctor Fiorentino then explained he must take a biopsy from my elbow since that was required to confirm the diagnosis of dermatomyositis.

   I was administered a local numbing and he took a deep biopsy at the point of elbow. It was painful.

4. Doctor Fiorentino then discussed the likely sequence of treatment and the drugs that would be involved. Most of this did not register with me, I was overwhelmed by events, and I had to rely on the notes of Aurdery to recall that it even happened.

5. After this thorough examination and much discussion, they continued my prescription of 80 gm/day of prednisone plus all the other medications prescribed by Doctor Austin.

They then provided a brief description of the disease and what it meant to me. They explained it usually occurs as a result of a cancer somewhere in the body, so they scheduled examinations to explore this possibility, including a CAT scan, colonoscopy, follow-up examinations at the Digestive Health Clinic, function tests at the Pulmonary Clinic, endocrine ultra sound of pancreas, and a thorough skin dermatology examination. These all occurred over the next two months; after these exhausting examinations they reached the conclusion that I was cancer-free. [14]

Wow! I was eighty years of age with no apparent cancer anywhere – that result was pleasing - maybe – then I remembered I did have a serious, incurable disease.

This first encounter with the team was an overwhelming experience. Dr. Fiorentino asked: "did I have any questions?" Yes, enough to fill a book, but I could only focus on the priorities at the moment: "Is the disease treatable? What is my prognosis? What happens next?"

His responses seemed vague, and rightly so. He offered hope and encouragement but tempered it by telling me there was a range of experience with different people. The outlook for successful treatment was good and we would start today. He told me there were several medications available for treatment. He mentioned IVIG, whatever that was. He explained the biopsy was necessary because blood tests by themselves were not definitive. He asked me for the name of my pharmacy in Sonora and said all my prescriptions would be sent there. I was scheduled for my next appointment in another month, recognizing that I lived in Sonora, a four hour road trip away. He then asked me to continue to utilize my Sonora family physician for all the usual medical issues while he dealt with the new disease.

---

[14] A cancer was to be discovered seven years later in the form of Multiple Myeloma, a cancer of plasma cells, a type of white blood cell normally responsible for producing antibodies.

Also a member of the team was Dr. Chung, a Professor of Medicine (Immunology, Rheumatology, and Dermatology) at Stanford University School of Medicine. This inter-discipline team was able to bring to bear the latest expertise relative to immune diseases.

For the past seven years, I have had an examination every three months with Dr. Fiorentino and his team at the Stanford Health Clinic. He examined the status of my rash and muscles. In addition to these complete examinations, he also reviewed the ongoing treatment and any changes. After the seven years of treatment, my maintenance of the disease is stable.

5

SPOUSE AND FAMILY

Thank God for the support of my wife and children; without them, I could not have made it emotionally through the long ordeal. As a patient with a serious disease, you do not suffer alone. Your family is equally affected and, perhaps, even more so as they make the necessary adjustments to a new lifestyle that was not in their game plan. You have little choice about what transpires, but they do. If you are fortunate, as I was, they will willingly and gracefully accept the new privations. You should not take their accommodation or their sacrifices for granted, but acknowledge and respond in a positive manner.

Let me relate one example. Early on with the disease when my muscle strength was at low ebb, practically non-existent, I decided to take a bath, filled the tub, and lay on my back submerged. When it was time to push myself up from the water, I found my muscles so weak I was unable to do this. Calling my wife, I asked her to help lift me up to a sitting position. She was unable to accomplish this. I told her to go to the garage, get a small plank and insert it under my shoulders, which she did. After a struggle, she helped me from the bathtub. It was a wakeup call for both of us that we had to become a two-person team.

During all the seven years she has accompanied me on the four-hour car trip from Sonora to the Stanford Hospital in Palo Alto and waited in the hospital or elsewhere for the three days of my IVIG treatments, and then endured the four-hour road trip back to Sonora. She never complained about the inconvenience and tried to turn it into a positive, which made my own medical requirements easier to accept.

During the initial office visit with the team, the subject arose: "Did I want to be placed in their research program?"

The answer for me was clear. My grandson had already been successfully treated at the Stanford Children's' hospital for Leukemia in a research program and I had been educated by his mother, my daughter. I felt I may receive better care under the controlled conditions of a research program with the availably of new types of treatments or medications, not otherwise available to me. There would be an information fire-wall erected between what I needed to know for successful treatment, and what I could not be told about research results. I could opt out at any time but the exit would be a one-way street.

My answer to Doctor Fiorentino was: "yes, I wanted to be in the research program."

6

MEDICATIONS

From earliest days I have always had access to good health care. Even in the rural, impoverished region of South Dakota during the 1930's Great Depression our family was able to utilize a doctor appointed as the county health care doctor to supply our medical needs. As a consequence, I have always availed myself of whatever resources were appropriate for maintaining good health. During later careers as naval officer and business executive, I continued to follow the medical advice of my family doctor.

When I became ill with dermatomyositis, I followed this lifelong pattern and embraced the best medical available, which was that provided by the specialized team at the Stanford Health Care clinic at Redwood City.

*M*edications perform a vital and almost the only significant role in treating dermatomyositis. It is with use of medications that a person can survive and even obtain a reasonably satisfactory quality-of-life. There is virtually no other means of treatment than through the use of various medications and infusions.

The following are a few comments about some of the principle medications utilized during my treatment. I will start with a discussion of two early-on medications normally utilized that ultimately proved unsatisfactory for my treatment: azathioprine and methotrexate.

(a). Azathioprine was first used in 1957 and has been approved by the FDA as an immunosuppressive medication used in rheumatoid arthritis and in kidney transplants to prevent rejection. Other medical uses are considered "off label", but it has been employed in immune suppressant therapy for other diseases. Before the development of Cellcept that came later, the medication most commonly used in prior years for treating dermatomyositis was azathioprine. It was a troublesome medication and not always effective or tolerated by many patients. Diarrhea, nausea, and vomiting were common problems. Other serious risk factors include an increased risk of lymphoma. It is listed by the International Agency for Research on Cancer as a group 1 carcinogen (carcinogenic to humans). [15]

Shortly after starting treatment with Azathioprine, I developed a major diarrhea problem, became ill, entered the Stanford Hospital emergency ward, and was immediately taken off this medication.

---

[15] "Azathioprine", Wikipedia, 2017

(b). <u>Methotrexate</u> is a chemotherapy agent and immune system suppressant also typically used in treating this disease. It is used to treat cancer, autoimmune diseases, and for medical abortions. Types of cancers it is used for include breast cancer, leukemia, lung cancer, and lymphoma. Types of autoimmune diseases it is used for include psoriasis, rheumatoid arthritis, and Crohn's disease. [16]

Common side effects include nausea, feeling tired, fever, increased risk of infection, and low white blood cell counts. Other side effects may include liver disease, lung disease, lymphoma, and severe skin rashes. People on long-term treatment should be regularly checked for side effects. Methotrexate initially came into medical use to treat cancer, as it was less toxic than the other treatments used at that time. [17]

Methotrexate was prescribed for me as a replacement of the Azathioprine. It was a drug developed for use in suppressing the immune system. It seemed to be reasonably effective in treating my disease, but it does have the downside of a tendency to lead to infections. That was the result for me and three month after beginning its use, I developed pneumonia, and was immediately taken off the medication.

I was placed on several other drugs (on a research basis) to find the one best suited to me. A *Hydrocyelclor* trial began on

---

[16] "Methotrexate", Wikipedia, 2017

[17] ibid

10/18/2011, but was stopped because of diarrhea. During that year I was also given a <u>Rituxan</u> treatment on a research basis to see if it was of benefit, but the results were inconclusive.

One of the advantages of being on a research program, as I was, is for the trial of various medications and treatments under carefully controlled conditions to determine if there are better alternatives. The end result of these trials in my case was that the best medication choices for me were Cellcept, immunoglobulin (IVIG), and prednisone.

> (c). <u>Prednisone</u>. This is a corticosteroid medication that is a steroid, and is often the preferred method of treatment. Prednisone is particularly effective as an immune-suppressant drug. It is used to treat certain inflammatory diseases, autoimmune diseases, and some types of cancer, but it has significant adverse effects. [18]

The mechanism of action for prednisone is to improve renal responsiveness by increasing the density of peptide receptors in the renal inner collecting duct, inducing a potent dieresis. [19] (I do not fully understand this complex medical language, but I accept the results.)

For some people especially children, symptoms may resolve

---

[18] "Prednisone", Wikipedia, 2017

[19] Ibid

completely after a treatment with corticosteroids. This is called remission. It is seldom achieved with adults. [20]

Corticosteroids (prednisone) shouldn't be used for long periods of time because of their potential side effects. I was on prescriptions of prednisone for nearly seven years and it contributed to the onset of my type-two diabetic condition. (I was already insulin resistant before beginning its use.) I was initially placed on 80mg/day in the local Sonora hospital, which was quickly lowered during subsequent treatment to 60mg/day, then later to 15mg/day for several years. The doctor will most likely start with a high dose and then gradually lower it with dosage dependent on what appears to be needed. [21]

Prednisone can become somewhat addictive. To ween me off of it after six years, I started at 10 mg/day and gradually reduced it by 1 mg/day over a several week period before I was able to stop it entirely. I no longer utilize prednisone or feel the need of it in my treatment. [22]

(d). *Mycophenolic acid (Cellcept):* is the major medication employed over a period of six years for my daily treatment. It is an immuno-suppressant drug marketed under the trade name Cellcept. It was first approved by the FDA in 1995 for use in kidney transportation and since then

---

[20] ibid

[21] ibid

[22] ibid

utilized for other organs such as the heart, liver, and lung. It inhibits an enzyme needed for the growth of T cells and B cells. [23]

Before the development of Cellcept, the medication most commonly used in prior years was azathioprine. It was a troublesome medication and not always effective or tolerated by many patients. Diarrhea was a common problem. Cellcept has a lower incidence of diarrhea with no increase in the risk or any of the other side effects. [24] I take three Cellcept tablets every morning and two every night an hour before consuming food; each capsule is 500mg, 2500mg/day, which is a powerful drug treatment.

A downside of Cellcept is its cost. It is 15 times more expensive than azathioprine. The exact role of mycophenolate-vs-azathioprine has yet to be conclusively established, which is, perhaps, an objective of the current research. [25]

The use of the Cellcept medication in my treatment of dermatomyositis is an "off label" use, which is permitted as a result of my participation in a research program to determine if it will assist the immune system in mitigating the action of attacking the skin and muscles. I am most fortunate to be in the research program that permits the use of this medication on a research

---

[23] "Mycophenolic Acid", Wikipedia, 2017

[24] ibid

[25] ibid

basis that has been successful during most of the seven years of my treatment.

> (e). <u>IVIG (Immunoglobulin therapy).</u> This IVIG medication treatment is an I V infusion of immunoglobulin that has been utilized in my treatment of dermatomyositis for six years.

IVIG (immunoglobulin therapy) first occurred in the 1930s and injection into a vein was approved for medical use in the United States in 1981. Immunoglobulin therapy is used in a variety of conditions, many of which involve decreased antibody production capability. It is used in many autoimmune disorders such as dermatomyositis in an attempt to decrease the severity of symptoms.[26]

A human body with the disease is producing antibodies that target skin and muscles and an infusion of intravenous immuno-globulin uses healthy antibodies to block these harmful antibodies. I have been receiving this IVIG treatment on a cycle of every six or eight weeks on three consecutive days at the Stanford Hospital's Ambulatory Infusion Center now for seven years.

IVIG consists of a mixture of antibodies that have been collected from thousands of healthy people who have donated their blood. These antibodies are given to the patient through an IV infusion.

---

[26] "IVIG", Wikipedia 2017

This is a procedure with me sitting in a chair getting the IV infusion on three consecutive days on a cycle every six or eight weeks. A nurse inserts an intravenous needle into a vein in my arm and the infusion begins that lasts four or five hours. I am given pre-medications of Tylenol and Benadryl. The infusion is essentially painless following the premedication and sometimes I doze.

In finding a vein and getting a needle into it that is more fragile because of my advanced age and the prednisone, the nurses always found my veins a difficult medical challenge. This procedure began with them hunting for a suitable vein somewhere on my lower arm. I could never see any veins, but with much tapping up and down my arm to cause the veins to rise, they finally locate a suitable one and began the sterile medical procedure for pushing a needle through the skin and inside the vein. There were often several attempts at insertion into a vein before success and I learned to live with many needle pokes.

I soon became acquainted with the four nurses in attendance in the Infusion Center. They handled as many as a dozen patients at a time in the three four-person treatment modules of the Center. I developed an appreciation for their expertise in handling the wide variety of patients, who often had as many as a dozen different kinds of bags of infusion medications hanging from overhead being fed into their veins. Each patient had a different set of orders from their own doctors with treatment instructions for their particular disease.

I often wondered about the wide range of ailments each was being treated for. I saw few bags of the same size, shape, and color of medication as mine, but I never felt it was appropriate for me to ask about the illness of others.

OTHER MEDICAL CONDITIONS AND DRUGS: I had also been given prescriptions in previous years for various other medical conditions.

Scurvy: When I was in graduate school at Berkeley and living an unhealthy lifestyle and eating nothing but hamburgers, I developed a bad breath. Since I was in the active naval reserve, I went to the reservist naval dentist on my drill night at Treasure Island. He asked me questions about my activities and menu, looked in my mouth, and told me the reason for my bad breath was a case of borderline scurvy. At his prompting, I began taking vitamin C, a multivitamin, and improved my diet to include fresh fruit. My bad breath was cured within a week. That was in 1956, and I am still taking vitamin C and a multivitamin 60 years later. Apparently I had susceptibility for the problems of scurvy. When I find something that solves a problem and works, I stick with it.

Hypertension (high blood pressure): Dr. Austin made the diagnosis of a borderline hypertension condition fifteen years ago and placed me on prescriptions for Atenolol and Lisinopril.

Type Two Diabetes: For several years I had lived with a condition of borderline insulin resistance. I gradually developed type two diabetes as a result of taking Prednisone for a long period of time;

so, I was given prescriptions for Glimepiride and Janumet to treat the diabetes.

Gout: as a result of uric acid that has always bordered on the high side (a tendency inherited from my mother), I take Colchicine when needed to head-off a painful gout attack.

Statin: I have been prescribed Lipitor for a number of years as a preventative to maintain my cholesterol at acceptable low levels.

Other conditions: I also take preventative over-the-counter pills including vitamin D, vitamin C, vitamin B12(for anemia), and a multivitamin (Centrum Silver). As early as 1960, I began taking a daily aspirin when I became convinced it was truly beneficial. The American Medical Association finally realized the same thing a dozen years later.

Drugs for Multiple Myeloma: I will discuss this major addition to my drug regimen in a later chapter on this disease.

My Rules for taking pills: I take twenty medications per day. Most of these are prescription but also a number of others are vitamins, with half of the pills taken in the morning and the other half in the evening. This places considerable stress on my stomach and it is important to avoid upsets to my digestive system. I have a simple rule: always follow a session of pill-taking with a bite of food and glass of milk. The only exception to this is with Cellcept, which requires taking it on an empty stomach at least an hour before eating any food.

Fortunately I have a "cast-iron" stomach because I have never had any upset as a result taking all this medication.

At an appropriate time during a person's life, the use of medications becomes necessary to maintain optimal health with advancing age when some organs become less efficient or with the onset of disease. Some of these are available as over-the-counter pills but others require a prescription to obtain. I attribute the effective use of medications with helping me maintain reasonably satisfactory health despite several diseases.

Here is a list of my medications and what each is for.

1. Scurvy 1951. Vitamin C and multi-vitamin. Bad breath caused by improper diet in Graduate School at U.C, Berkeley. Continued to present day.

Vit. C	500/day	1 tab/day
Multi-Vit.	1 Tab/day	

2. Hypertension 2000. Dr. Austin & Dr. Allen

Atenolol 50mg.	2 tab/day
Lisinopril 20mg.	1 tab/day
Amlopipine 5 mg.	1 tab/day

3. Type Two Diabetes. 2011 Dr. Austin & Dr. Allen

Glimepiride 4 mg.	2 tab/day
Janumet 50mg-500mg.	2 tab/day

4. Dermatomyositis. 2010 Dr. Fiorentino, Stanford

Cellcept 500mg.	5 tab/day
IVIG.	Immune Goblin 180 gr.
	3 days every 8 weeks
Folic Acid 1 mg.	1 tab/day
Prednisone 15mg. 1 tab/day	(no long utilized)
Calcium +Vit. D 1000mg.	1 tab/day

5. Multiple Myeloma. 2017 Dr. Iberri, Stanford

Revlimid (Lenalidomide) 15mg.	for 21 day/month
1 tab/day	
Dexamethasone 4mg.	5 tab/week all at once
Zometa IV infusion	1/month
Aspirin 87mg.	2 tab/day

6. High cholesterol Dr. Austin

Lipitor 40mg	1 tab/day

7. Gout. High level of uric acid. Dr. Austin & Dr. Allen

Colchicine 0.6mg. Daily or as needed for pain

8. Anemic Dr. Allen

Vit. B 12	1000 IU	1tab/day

9. Insufficient Sun Dr. Allen

Vit. D3	1000IU	1 tab/day

Wow! That is a lot of medication. I have questioned my Internist, Dr. Allen, if all the prescriptions are still appropriate, and the answer is yes.

As a means of managing my medications, plus those taken by my wife, Aurdery, I utilize five seven-day pill boxes, three for me and two for Aurdery, with one for each morning and one for the evening. I refill the pill boxes each week and check to determine if I need to reorder any medications. Managing the medications is an important job and I find the use of pill boxes to be absolutely necessary.

7

MEDICAL EXPERTISE

I have now had several years of first-hand exposure and experience with several doctors at the Stanford Medical Hospital and Clinics, and locally here in Sonora; so, permit me to comment on what they all seem to have in common.

First of all, they all have a high IQ to deal with the complexities of medical science, second is a scientific curiosity to identify what makes things happen, and third is a genuine effort to provide a medical service to others.

After Dr. Austin retired, I was fortunate to obtain the services of another local internist for my personal physician, Dr. David Allen. He received his training at the Loma Linda College in Southern California. Inasmuch as his resume is not as long or impressive on paper as that of Dr. Austin, I rate him as an excellent physician, and I am fortunate to receive his medical services.

I was also fortunate to receive the referral to Dr. David Fiorentino MD., Ph.D. who was the medical expert in charge of my treatment for dermatomyositis. In addition to teaching in the Stanford School of Medicine, he is also the leading hands-on practitioner in the clinic where patients are under his care. He is a Professor in the Department of Dermatology and Department of Immunology and Rheumatology at Stanford University School of Medicine. He completed his M.D. and Ph.D. degrees at Stanford University. Dr. Fiorentino has served as the Co-Director of the multidisciplinary Rheumatology-Dermatology clinic that has been in operation at Stanford since 2003. His research interests focus on rheumatic skin diseases such as dermatomyositis, scleroderma, and lupus; hence, he is both a teacher and a hands-on clinical practitioner of medicine involving immune diseases.

Lorinda Chung MD MS is Associate Professor of Medicine (Immunology and Rheumatology) and Dermatology at Stanford University School of Medicine. Dr. Chung initiated and developed the Stanford Scleroderma Center of Excellence.

I was fortunate to have these highly trained medical experts locally in Sonora and at Stanford Hospital in assisting with my care.

8

DIGESTIVE HEALTH

It was no small thing that I was referred to the Digestive Health Clinic at the onset of my new disease. The medical staff had already recognized that my digestive system would encounter problems with inadequate muscle strength - and it did. The digestive system also operates like other parts if the body with motive power controlled by a complexity of muscles and chemicals such as juices supplied by the pancreas.

Within days of my new illness I encountered frequent episodes of constipation and diarrhea. I alternated between taking over-the-counter medications of a laxative for constipation followed by Imodium to deal with diarrhea, one condition followed by the other.

The condition in which the muscles throughout my body were weakened included interior muscles such as those that control my digestive system and caused a lack of control of my bowel movements. The thirty feet of intestines, colon, and rectum all function with the help of internal muscles that help propel and control the contents. I frequently (nearly every day) had sudden and unanticipated bowel movements with only a couple seconds advance warning - sometimes not enough time to reach the toilet (and I have three toilets in the house). I quickly opted for throw-away underwear.

The episodes became unpleasant occurrences that placed great stress on day-to-day activities. I never learned fully how to deal with the problem, but it gradually improved as medications provided better control of my internal digestive muscles. As suggested by the Digestive Health Clinic I began to take a daily stool softener pill and increased my intake of fiber.

I have become an advocate of bidets. In my international business travels I had often encountered the bidets that were in evidence alongside toilet stools in Europe, particularly in France. The Sonora residence I purchased had a bidet already installed in the master bathroom alongside the toilet stool, but I ignored it and it remained unused for several years. Then I developed a problem with hemorrhoids as a result of constipation and read where hot water baths from a bidet were useful. That led me into a daily use of our bidet. Since then I have utilized our bidet on a daily basis.

The pancreas is a glandular organ in the digestive and endocrine system that is located in the abdominal cavity behind the stomach. It produces several important hormones which circulate in the blood, including insulin and glucagon. The pancreas secrets juices containing digestive enzymes that assist digestion and absorption of nutrients in foods in the small intestine. These enzymes help to further break down carbohydrates, proteins, and lipids. In addition to supplying insulin, the pancreas also provides digestive juices that help in the process of digestion.

The pancreas is a difficult organ to observe from outside the body because of its location behind the stomach, so obtaining effective information from outside through the skin is somewhat ineffective. For that reason, a patient must swallow a device that travels into the stomach and is positioned where it can make an echo sound of the pancreas through the wall of the stomach. That test of the endocrine system was conducted in the Digestive Health Clinic of Stanford. The results indicated a normal pancreas, a relief for me since my brother had died of pancreatic cancer.

Perhaps the most important service provided for me by the Digestive Health Clinic was to emphasize the importance of a proper diet that included adequate fiber.

9

PULMONARY ISSUES

Dr. Fiorentino insisted I avail myself of a Function Test each year in the Pulmonary Clinic as a means to determine that all my pulmonary organs (lungs and bronchial passageways) remained in good health. Side effects as the result of my illness were often pulmonary problems. The incidence of COPD (Chronic Obstructive Pulmonary Disease) is the third leading cause of death in the United States behind heart issues and cancer; so, it was important to monitor this condition.

The functional tests in the Pulmonary Clinic are rather simple. The principle one has the name of Spirometry and consists of blowing into a mouthpiece. That does not seem very sophisticated, but the volume and composition of the exhaust air is chemically analyzed in a number of different ways and catalogued by computer control. Over time, the results can provide a good measure of the condition of the pulmonary system. Following this spirometry test, the patient conducts a five-minute walk with all the vital components measured before and after the exertion. Those two hands-on tests provide an assessment of the patient's pulmonary system. If any deficiencies are found, a CAT scan is performed to identify the problem areas.

Fortunately for me, my pulmonary system was in excellent shape. Perhaps my most important personal contributions were no smoking for the past fifty years and a rigorous exercise program.

10

EXERCISE AND LIFE ADMUSTMENTS

Perhaps you are becoming bored with all this discussion about medical problems and issues; if so, join the party. So am I. The difference between you and me is that you can close the book and go do something else, but I do not have that luxury. These are things I have to deal with each and every day if I want to continue to enjoy a reasonable quality-of-life. Take exercise, for example. I have been a strong advocate for strenuous aerobic exercise on a daily basis and I still continue to try to do it as best I can.

From earliest childhood, I have always been physically active. During the 1930's living in the small rural town of Buffalo Gap, we kids were in motion from morning to night. During high school, I was on every football, basketball, and track team in addition to numerous jobs and chores. As adults, our family participated in numerous physical activities such as swimming, hiking, fishing, and tennis. We engaged in these things because it was part of our way-of-life. We never considered that we were engaging in "exercise"; we were just having fun.

After I retired, my wife and I joined a sport and recreation facility to obtain the regular exercise we both realized we needed. We maintained excellent physical condition during our retirement years.

The discovery that I had an autoimmune disease, dermatomyositis, came as a shock. I have now been under successful treatment for many years and I attribute much of the success of my treatment to the physical condition of my body at the onset of the disease and maintaining a reduced exercise regimen since that time appropriate for my disease.

The websites that discussed dermatomyositis were somewhat mixed on the subject of exercise – yes do it, or no, avoid physical activity – a jumbled message. As an advocate of strenuous aerobic exercise, I made the personal decision that I would continue to engage in it to the extent possible. As a consequence, during the past seven years of my disease, I have engaged in twenty-minutes of an exercise routine every morning before my shower. I begin with the eye muscles, neck muscles, arms, legs, and gradually work down to my toes, working every muscle in my body. My muscles have never atrophied. I am convinced that some of the success of my treatment is the result of this daily exercise program.

When a person engages in vigorous exercise, he (or she) causes the blood to pump through every nook and cranny of the body.

Every muscle and organ receives the oxygen from the red blood cells that flow through the blood stream; hence, no part of the body is deprived of this life-giving oxidation. That is true not only for the arms and legs but also for the brain, pancreas, internal muscles of the intestines and rectum and neglected areas such as the toes and fingertips. Exercise is a magic tonic for the entire body.

11

ACCOMODATIONS, FAMILY SPACES, AND MOTELS

My home in Sonora is located within a mile of the excellent hospital, Adventist Healthcare, and I also have as my local family doctor an internist physician who gives me excellent medical care. But, the treatment of some diseases requires the use of specialists; therefore, I welcomed the advice from my family doctor, Dr. Austin, to seek a referral to the Immunology Team at Stanford Hospital who specialized in my disease.

Stanford Hospital in Palo Alto is located in the center of Silicon Valley, one of the busiest and most expensive real estate markets in the nation. The cost of motels reflects the business climate in which thousands of computer and technical people are vying for motel reservations. Costs are sky-high.

Fortunately for me, my daughter and family live in Palo Alto and when I first started my treatment they had a spare room available to me, so I was able temporarily to escape the high cost of motels. That was later to change. It raises the issue of what accommodations to utilize when you must travel and stay at a hospital or clinic far from where you live?

The costs involved are no small matter. In Silicon Valley at the present time, a night's stay on a Friday or Saturday night at a Holiday Inn or equivalent will cost in the range of $175 -$200/night. That same room during week nights when all the businessmen on expense accounts descend on the area will cost upwards of $300.

How many people with a serious disease who must arrange accommodations for a spouse or family member can afford those kinds of costs?

I was financially better prepared because of a long career as a business executive that enabled me to build a nest egg; hence, I was temporarily able to handle the penalty of the high costs involved. That is not the case for everyone. What is someone to do who finds themselves needing the medical care of an institution far removed from home? The options will vary and there are no pat answers. I was unable to find other rooming opportunities in the Bay Area, and perhaps there were better or cheaper alternatives than those I utilized.

Some medical costs do permit a tax offset, but these are limited. Medical costs are limited to those above 7.5% of Adjusted Gross Income, so they do not kick-in until they become substantial. Meals are limited to $20/day and lodging to $100/night, so these allowances are inadequate to cover the actual costs.

It is unfortunate but true, that at the same time a person faces the high cost of medications and health care, he or she may also encounter the high cost of travel and accommodations.

12

ELDERLY DRIVING AND RULES-OF-THE-ROAD

I must travel from my home in Sonora every other month the 150 miles to Stanford Hospital for my three days of IVIG treatment in addition to other office visits in Palo Alto. That is a four-hour one-way trip that carries my auto over 50 miles of a winding two-lane country road-, another 50 miles after I join the 6-lane commuting crowd of autos heading to the Bay Area, and then another 50 miles of Bay Area freeways that are some of the most crowded and challenging freeways in the nation. Then I have to travel it in the reverse direction after my medical appointments are completed. It is not an auto trip designed for an amateur driver or for the faint-hearted.

I have now successfully managed this travel challenge for a number of years, and face it at the age of 88. How do I manage to accomplish it? It requires discipline, and here is my "rules-for-the-road."

1. When I must leave in the very early morning (6am), I always arise early and spend two hours getting myself fully energized and emotionally ready to take the trip. I shower, have coffee for the caffeine, and a small breakfast for nourishment.

2. I utilize the speed control in my auto and religiously follow the speed limits. The only exception to this occurs when I am in heavy traffic and must go-with-the-flow. Attempting to go slower than the flow is to invite the dangerous practice of tailgating.

3. Many serious accidents occur because of improper lane changes. To the extent possible, I always attempt to stay in my own lane whenever possible. I attempt to maintain an awareness of other divers behind or alongside me, but in the heavy multi-lane traffic of the Bay Area freeways that is often unrealistic; therefore, I always use considerable caution in changing lanes. Prior to changing into another lane to my right, I <u>always</u> glance over my right shoulder to insure that lane is safely available, and in changing into a lane on my left, I do the same over the left shoulder. Every few seconds I glance at my rear view mirror to see who is behind me. I also use my side mirrors, but have found they often have blind spots, hence, the glance over-the-shoulder. This simple procedure of a quick glance over a shoulder has saved me from a major lane-change accident at least once

every year. Maybe it is over-kill, but I am not prepared to accept that one accident.

4. I will drive after I become tired as a matter of necessity, but I <u>never</u> drive if I become sleepy. The way to avoid sleep when driving is a simple matter of developing the proper discipline. When I was a naval officer in combat, to sleep on duty was a serious court martial offense, so I learned discipline. When driving a car, sleep can become a death sentence. I consider drifting into the habit of sleep extremely serious and give it the high priority the matter deserves. Driving wide-awake is a matter of discipline.

5. I have found several means of reducing stress during driving: caffeine, chewing gum, and having background music on my satellite radio. I usually stop at a McDonalds in Tracy at the half-way point after two hours for a brief change of pace. I go to the restroom, get my body moving again, and have a coffee.

During my first trip to the Bay Area after my diagnosis seven years ago, I received a speeding ticket. I had to go to traffic school to avoid a cost penalty on my insurance. That ticket and traffic school was one of the fortunate things to happen to me. I immediately decided to change my over-aggressive and sloppy driving habits and start utilizing my rules-for-the-road. In the years since then, I have enjoyed driving more and have now become a much better driver. In fact, at 88 years-of-age, I am a better driver than I was ten years ago.

13

PROMPT CARE AND EMERGENCY WARD

The local Sonora Adventist Care hospital maintains a Prompt Care facility for the use of people who need this temporary means of medical attention available on short notice. My family and I have utilized it many times. In my own case, I received a diagnosis of pneumonia several years ago that was timely and important for my recovery. My wife also received a diagnosis and treatment for pneumonia. One visiting son with a lingering cold he was ignoring, who I encouraged to go to Prompt Care, received a diagnosis of pneumonia. Another visiting son from New York received a diagnosis of Lime Disease that he had contacted in New York and was given the necessary medication to avoid potentially serious medical issues. My family and I utilize this facility on short notice whenever needed.

In addition to utilizing Prompt Care, I also have gone to the Emergency Ward of our local Adventist Hospital on several occasions. Like many others, I have a tendency when feeling ill to procrastinate and wait too long before seeking proper medical attention. I have now learned that some conditions are not likely to go away or improve without medical help, so am now more inclined to act when a problem is in the early stages. During the past year, I have twice gone to the Emergency Ward in the middle of the night to deal with a medical problem that could not wait for the morning. In each instance, I prevented a more serious problem and immediately received the expertise medical treatment I needed.

14

ATTITUDE

Pain is a symptom of an underlying condition. [27] The presence of cancer pain depends mainly on the location of the cancer and the stage of the disease. At any given time, two thirds of those with advanced cancer experience pain of such intensity that it adversely affects their sleep, mood, social relations and activities of daily living. [28]

One of the most important factors in dealing with cancer is attitude: how to deal emotionally with pain and the other trappings (such as medications) that come with the territory. Feeling sorry for oneself is an easy pitfall that only magnifies the problems.

There are several ways to keep a positive attitude. Dr. Norman Vincent Peal, a well-known guru of sixty five years ago in his famous book: *The Power of Positive Thinking*, dealt with it in a

---

[27] "Pain", Wikipedia, 2017

[28] ibid

religious way: "Why not draw upon that Higher Power." [29] If you believe in the Christian God like Dr. Peal, then a religious approach and prayer may work for you and if so, then you are fortunate to have a religious faith to help you.

If, however, you are an atheistic, like half the people in the world, then you must approach an illness and its suffering in a secular and more philosophical manner. There are no proven means to do this, and each must find their own way.

Personally, I only worry about those things I can actually control. If it is something I have absolutely no control over, then why worry about it? Accept it for what it is, and move on to something else you can actually control. If your genome is a cause of an illness, which is unfortunate but maybe the luck of the draw; accept it, and then muster the best resources available to deal with it. Perhaps in hindsight you could have done things differently in avoidance, but there is little to be gained in personal recrimination after the fact.

It is important to keep your self-confidence and avoid the despondency that can develop with negative news. Let me give a personal example. On a recent trip to Palo Alto I avoided the intake of water so I could make the four-hour trip without stopping for a pee break. On arrival at the hospital I took a blood test in a dehydrated condition. In the following review with the doctor

---

[29] Norman Vincent Peal, The Power of Positive Thinking, Fawcett Crest books, NY, 1952

I was shocked to learn my GFR reading (Glomerular Filtration Rate) was so low it indicated a serious kidney problem. The doctor ordered an immediate IV infusion of liquids. I became despondent that my efforts at personal control had led me into a kidney problem. A week later after the intake of fluids, I repeated the blood test and the GFR were again normal. My changing attitude reacting to news had led me into, and back out of the despondency that developed with negative news.

I will attempt to maintain a positive attitude about life, my quality-of-life, and accentuate the positive to the maximum extent I can. Please, wish me the luck-of-the-Irish.

15

MULTIPLE MYELOMA

"Cancer Center! Dad, you didn't tell me your appointment was at the cancer center."

"I guess I didn't realize it was," I responded, somewhat embarrassed. This was my third trip to this wing of the Stanford Hospital and the first time I looked up at the nameplate over the entrance and saw the words: CANCER CENTER.

My oldest daughter, Treci, accompanied me on the four-hour trip from Sonora. I drove the car this morning and she would drive tonight on the return trip. This was my third time to this clinic with endless tests: blood tests, CAT scan, 24 hour urine test, and bone marrow biopsy. Now it was crunch time and this appointment with Dr. Iberri, a specialist in hematology. I failed to realize the word "cancer" was involved. The rest of the day became a blur. Thank God that Treci was along to take notes.

Today was my eighty-eighth birthday and I was given the present of a new disease, multiple myeloma. Happy birthday, Bernie – welcome to your new world.

The word myeloma is from the Greek "myelo" meaning marrow, and "oma" meaning tumor. It is a cancer of the blood - the uncontrolled growth of abnormal plasma cells (a type of white blood cell). They become cancerous in the bone marrow and form multiple masses (tumors).

Plasma cells are white blood cells that normally secrete large volumes of antibodies to fight disease. They are transported by the blood plasma and lymph fluid in the immune system and originate in the bone marrow. Normally, once released into the blood stream and lymph fluid, these antibody molecules bind to the target antigen (foreign substance) and initiate its neutralization or destruction, but now I had the worst of the bad: runaway plasma cells.

Permit me to digress so you will understand the academic limitations that cloud my descriptions. In my long-ago college years, I studied inorganic chemistry. The structure of inorganic molecules made some sense to me at that time and I was able to utilize valences and the periodic table to actually understand inorganic chemical reactions (somewhat, enough to earn me a degree in physics).

Organic chemistry is a far-more complicated ballgame. It is like comparing Buffalo Gap to New York City; the added complexity is baffling. There seems to be little rhyme or reason to the structure of an organic molecule; so, now you understand my difficulty in trying to explain the organic chemistry of the immune system in language that is simple. Let me also caution you that one of the resource materials from my library that I utilized is the 1960 copy of Collier's Encyclopedia – only 58 years old? So, what else is new?

Before we talk about a bone marrow that has become cancerous, let's discuss the normal function of the body's immune system. We briefly addressed it in a previous chapter. Much is the same as discussed in that chapter, except that now we will deal with the additional element of cancer.

Until I encountered immune problems, I knew practically nothing about that complex system and confess it is still somewhat of a mystery to me. It is a difficult area for medical science to investigate because the marrow (where everything starts) is enclosed inside the confines of a bone, which (as a gross understatement) is a difficult area to study.

The bone marrow consists of a number of proteins (amino acids are the structural units that make up most proteins). [30] These proteins in the marrow are large, complex organic molecules that are often linked end-to-end in long chains (called polypeptides). These proteins perform a vast array of functions, including catalyzing metabolic reactions, DNA replication, responding to stimuli, and transporting molecules from one location to another. Proteins differ from one another primarily in their genome sequence that is controlled by the genes on their chromosomes; hence, the genetic

---

[30] "Amino Acids", Collier's Encyclopedia, 1960, vol. 16, p. 49

code determines the chemical structure of these proteins in the marrow. [31]

In a normal immune system, these proteins perform a number of tasks, but two are primary: they manufacture red blood cells (hemoglobin) and plasma cells.

The red blood cells formed in the marrow pass through the wall of the bone in passageways called microvascular exchange blood vessels. They enter the blood stream where they pick up oxygen in the lungs to carry it throughout the body and supply it to all the muscles that depend on the oxygen of red blood cells to function properly.

The plasma cells have a different mission than the red blood cells. They are (more or less) held in reserve in the marrow like storm troopers until they receive information that a foreign invader (bacterial infection or virus) is present somewhere in the body. At that point, the plasma cells pass through the vascular passageway in the wall of the bone, enter the blood stream, travel to the battle site, and attack the foreign invader. The remnants and debris of the battle between plasma cells and foreign invaders are absorbed by the lymphatic fluid and travel back through the lymphatic nodes to be discharged into the blood stream and head for filtration in the kidney.

This is an overly-simplified description of what routinely takes place in a normal immune system. Now let's look at what happens

[31] ibid

in the immune system for someone such as me who is inflicted with the autoimmune disease, dermatomyositis, as I have been for the past eight years.

Essentially everything happens the same way, except, (and it is a huge exception) the genes that determine the function and structure of the proteins in the marrow have been "corrupted" and cause the proteins in the marrow to misbehave. Instead of creating plasma cells that attack foreign invaders, the proteins create out-of-control freaks. These misguided plasma cells now see the body's own skin and muscles as foreign invaders, so attack them instead of the real enemy. That gives rise to the skin rashes and weakened muscles throughout the body.

I have described this as a battle of good guys –vs- bad boys, but in actually these are complex organic chemical reactions that occur as one molecule comes into contact with another, and keep-in-mind that these are large molecules that often assemble into long chains that connect to each other end-to-end. The marrow inside bones is a crowded place.

The long term prognosis for dermatomyositis is illustrated by my own experience. I have now been successfully treated with the help of the expertise of Stanford Medicine for eight years and have benefited from a reasonably satisfactory quality-of-life.

Now we will discuss the autoimmune disease that now threatens my life: multiple myeloma. Let's not kid ourselves; it is a horrific disease with painful experiences and a prognosis that no one wants to hear. After suffering the ravages of the disease that attack several of a person's vital organs, many people ultimately die of bone pain, pneumonia, kidney disease, or simply waste-away.

Multiple myeloma is a cancer of plasma cells, a type of white blood cell normally responsible for producing antibodies to fight infections. In the early stages, initial symptoms are often unnoticed or misdiagnosed. When it becomes advanced, bone pain, bleeding, frequent infections, anemia, and other onerous symptoms may occur. The prognosis becomes dire, depending on progression of the disease and the treatments available. [32]

The cause is generally unknown. [33] The protein in the bone marrow that normally produces plasma cells has undergone some sort of change due to a mutation in its controlling gene, or perhaps because of a structural abuse caused by some unknown influence or behavior. This protein undergoes chemical change and begins to produce plasma cells many times normal. The result is a glob of unstructured ex-protein that forms a mass, or several masses within the marrow, in what the medical profession refers to as a cancerous tumor. The tumor brings to a halt the normal functions of this protein in the marrow. As a consequence, several things happen simultaneously or progressively: the protein undergoes change; the plasma cells crowd out sufficient room for red blood cells leading to anemia; some of the tail-end chains become

---

[32] "Multiple Myeloma", Wikipedia, 2017

[33] ibid

particles unconnected to their host protein; the altered proteins cause a tumor mass that clogs the marrow; these protein chains begin to disintegrate as free light chain particles and pass through the vascular passageway into the blood, creating an overly thick blood that impedes and clogs blood flow; and the protein particles and free light chains in the blood stream create filtering problems that damage the kidney and cause kidney disease.

Wow! Some of that can occur even before you become aware of symptoms; so, a person can belatedly receive a diagnosis of the disease and begin treatment almost too late, already behind the eight ball.

Dr. Iberri was a young, knowledgeable, exceedingly sharp specialist with an excellent patient approach, and he laid-out an undisputable diagnosis: the blood and urine tests were consistent with the disease, the CAT scan had found bone lesions, and the bone marrow biopsy results confirmed the presence of cancer in the marrow. Treci recorded the facts and asked appropriate questions; I listened in a virtual fog.

Dr. Iberri explained the disease. For reasons unknown, the proteins in the marrow that normally produce healthy plasma cells become corrupted and begin to multiply rapidly in a runaway manner. It is not known why this happens, but one possible reason is a mutation in the genome on the chromosomes that control the proteins as a result of x-ray bombardment. These high energy x-ray jolts can change the makeup of genes, creating a mutation that leads to a different outcome. During my lifetime I have had dozens (perhaps hundreds) of these x-rays, CAT scans, MRIs, and related procedures, plus I also had exposure to radioactivity and atomic bomb tests as a naval officer.

Another cause may be indicated by the fact that the disease mostly attacks older people, suggesting that an age-related genome corruption or mutation may be a factor. Regardless of how it happened, these proteins in the marrow are altered and begin to produce plasma cells in a runaway fashion, far in excess of normal. This proliferation of plasma cells causes a tumor and is a blood cancer.

The cancerous plasma cells multiply so rapidly and begin to occupy such a large part of the marrow that they crowd out the red blood cells. That result was identified in blood tests that indicated the loss of hemoglobin and I was found to be anemic (insufficient number of red blood cells).

During the eight years of treatment for dermatomyositis, Dr. Fiorentino at the Stanford Medical Clinic prescribed blood tests every few months for monitoring my maintenance program. During the seventh year in 2017, he observed this pattern of a gradual decrease in the level of hemoglobin, indicating the onset of anemia and raised the question of "why"? This led him to the Hematology Clinic at the hospital where he contacted Dr. Iberri, a specialist in diseases related to blood. As a result of the alert by

Dr. Fiorentino and diagnosis by Dr. Iberri, I received an early diagnosis of the disease, which gave me better odds for treatment.

Before proceeding further, we need to understand what goes on in the marrow of the bone, which is the starting point for the immune system. Until I encountered immune problems, I knew practically nothing about that complex system and confess it is still somewhat of a mystery to me. It is a difficult area for medical science to study because the initial activity occurs in the marrow inside the bone.

The normal function of white blood cells once they are released into the blood and lymph is to bind with the target antigen (foreign substance) and initiate its neutralization or destruction. At least, that is what is supposed to happen in a healthy body, but the cancerous condition changes that. Multiple myeloma causes cancerous plasma cells to accumulate in the bone marrow where they crowd out healthy red blood cells, causing anemia. Rather than producing helpful antibodies, these cancerous cells cause a number of problems such as creating an inert mass of tumors in the bone marrow (definition of multiple myeloma), generating overly-thick blood that clogs blood flow, causing bone lesions that weaken bones throughout the body, bone pain (often manifest as the symptoms of a bad back), weakened bone conformation, uncontrolled infections, and protein remnants and free light chain particles that clog the kidney filtration process causing kidney problems or failure. (Wow – there are even more problems not listed here)

The prognosis is not favorable. In the United States it develops in 6.5 per 100,000 people per year and 0.7% of people are affected at some point in their life. It usually occurs around the age of 61 and is more common in men than women. Without treatment, typical survival is seven months. With current treatments, survival is about four years. [34]

Because many organs can be affected by myeloma, the symptoms vary greatly. A mnemonic sometimes used to remember some of the common symptoms of multiple myeloma is CRAB with: C = Calcium (elevated), R = Renal failure, A = Anemia, B = Bone lesions. Myeloma has many other possible symptoms, including opportunistic infections (e.g., pneumonia) and weight loss.

Now, let us look at some details involved with the disease.

Bone Pain:

Bone pain affects almost 70% of patients and is the most common symptom experienced by those afflicted with the disease. It is reportedly the cause of death in 30 % of those with the disease. [35]

Bone pain is pain originating from a bone (as differentiated from a muscle or other tissue). It occurs as a result of a wide range

---

[34] ibid

[35] "Reported on Yahoo," 7-13-2017

of causes and may severely impair the quality-of-life for patients who suffer from it. It arises in the periosteum, a membrane that covers the outer surface of all bones, except at the joints of long bones. [36] Bone pain is often experienced as a dull pain that cannot be localized accurately by the patient. This is in contrast with the traumatic pain that is suffered by the muscles or skin.

Bone plain usually involves the spine and ribs, and worsens with activity. Persistent localized pain may indicate a bone fracture, and involvement of the vertebrae may lead to spinal cord compression. The bone lesions observed in my initial CAT scan were lytic, meaning that soft spots develop where the bone structure has been damaged. These can extend from the inner bone marrow to the outside surface of the bone. These bone lesions weaken the bone, causing pain and increasing the risk of fractures. Bone loss frequently accompanies multiple myeloma, and 85% of patients diagnosed with the disease have some degree of bone loss. The breakdown of bone also leads to the release of calcium into the blood, leading to hypercalcemia and its associated symptoms.

Cause of bone pain:

It can have several possible causes ranging from extensive physical stress to serious diseases such as cancer. Bones are supplied with sensory neurons; yet, their exact anatomy remains obscure

---

[36] "Periosteal layer of bone tissue", Wikipedia, 2017

due to the contrasting physical properties of bone and neural tissue. The periosteal (sorry about using that obscure word) layer of bone tissue is highly pain-sensitive and an important cause of pain in several diseases like multiple myeloma. [37]

How is bone pain manifest in the patient:

Pain caused by cancer within bones is one of the most serious forms of pain because of its severity and uniqueness with respect to other forms of pain. It has been determined that bone pain related to cancer occurs as a result of destruction of bone tissue. Chemical changes that occur within the spinal cord as a result of bone destruction give further insight into the mechanism of bone pain. [38]

How to react to bone pain:

Control of pain with the use of over-the-counter medications such as Tylenol is seldom adequate and a prescription for pain medication is usually necessary.

The use of anesthetics within the actual bone has been a common treatment for several years. This method provides a direct approach using analgesics to relieve pain sensations. [39]

---

[37] "bone pain", Wikipedia, 2017

[38] ibid

[39] ibid

Physical activity can initiate bone pain and a patient must use care in the early stages to minimize this contribution. I have personally found that backing off from over-use of a body part when minor pain is first experienced and allowing it to fade away has been useful and sometimes even headed-off a further incident. For example: when a minor pain on my right shoulder was strong enough to interfere with my sleep, I slept on my left side and avoided all activity of my right shoulder for two weeks to the extent possible. The pain on the right shoulder suddenly disappeared and has not reoccurred.

That same tactic is more difficult to experience with lower back pain, but not completely. I do experience lower back pain. While still lying in bed, I spend a minute to exercise my body parts prior to placing weight on my legs

(I should do more of this but a have sudden need get out of bed and walk to the bathroom to urinate). For the first half hour, I use a cane and attempt to minimize pressure and activity on my lower back. The cane also provides stability support. My initial pain metric is about #3 or #4 (moderate). After slowly moving around on my feet for an hour, I find I no longer need the cane and can walk relatively pain free with a pain metric of #1 or #2 (zero to mild).

When shopping, I grab the nearest shopping cart in the parking lot to utilize as a walker in the store, which avoids the back strain from this activity. Then I observe other elderly shoppers walking in their stooped-over, hunched shuffle and know they could do a better job with their backs if they would utilize the resources avail to them. That is what I try to accomplish, not for purposes of image but for the health of my back. I am still too proud to utilize a rider cart during shopping, but that may be in my future.

I am not aware if the cause of my back pain is due to multiple myeloma, but assume it is. When laying in bed my spines becomes decompressed and then when standing the bone cartilages compress against each other, begin rubbing together, and create pain. The spaces between the vertebrae in my spine have shrunk during sleep. The more these spaces narrow and compress, the more likely the vertebrae are to encounter the spinal cord and the sensitive nerves that run up and down the center of each vertebrae. This can cause pressure on the nerve root itself, which is probably the point at which I start to experience back pain. [40]

There was no quick fix to back pain, but the more the activity the more likely the incidence and severity of pain. As a consequence, I force myself to sit down and take frequent periods of a sitting rest (and avoid lying on my back). My afternoon nap is accomplished in an easy chair in a sitting position. This rest procedure seems to work and the back pain level is now reasonably stabilized. [41]

---

[40] ibid

[41] "Bone pain", Wikipedia, 2017

Zometa:

As a preventive measure for bone weakness, I receive a monthly IV infusion of Zometa. Zoledronic acid with a trade name Zometa is a drug given intravenously to treat some bone diseases. Zometa is used to prevent skeletal fractures in patients with cancers such as multiple myeloma and prostate cancer as well as for treating osteoporosis. Zoledronic acid slows down bone resorption, allowing the bone-forming cells time to rebuild normal bone and allowing bone remodeling. [42]

Anemia:

The anemia found in myeloma usually results from the replacement of normal bone marrow by infiltrating tumor cells and inhibition of normal red blood cell production. This is normally found with a blood test indicating a lowering of hemoglobin, which is how my anemia was discovered. You may not feel any physical effects of anemia, but you become more vulnerable to infections.

Kidney failure:

The most common cause of kidney failure in multiple myeloma is due to protein fragments secreted by the malignant cells that

---

[42] "Zometa". Wikipedia. 2017

pass into the blood flow. Myeloma cells produce corrupted proteins, including particle fragments called free light chains. These proteins and particle fragments, depending on their size and makeup, can damage the filtering function of the kidney and cause kidney diseases.

The literature seems to understate the need for a steady consumption of liquids to promote the flow of protein contaminates in the blood stream through the kidney filtering process and their discharge in urination. I start my day with a glass of water taking my morning Cellcept, then two cups of coffee, followed with frequent consumption of milk, water, Gatorade, Diet Pepsi, and more water taken with my 10 pills in the morning and another 10 pills taken at night. I drink a lot of fluid throughout the day.

Infection:

The problem of fighting infections becomes a problem with the absence of effective plasma cells to fight infections. As already mentioned, the most common major infection encountered is pneumonia due to immune deficiency and kidney failure. Pneumonia is the most frequent cause of death. [43]

---

[43] ibid

Neurological symptoms:

Some symptoms (e.g., weakness, confusion, and fatigue) may be due to anemia; however, I am not aware of any of these issues. When the disease is well-controlled, neurological symptoms may result from treatments manifesting itself as numbness or pain in the hands, feet, and lower legs.

Risk factors:

The cause of multiple myeloma is generally unknown. Risk factors include drinking alcohol and obesity (but that can also be said for many diseases and is not specific to multiple myeloma). The underlying mechanism involves abnormal plasma cells producing abnormal antibodies, which form a tumor mass in the marrow. When more than one mass is formed, it is known as multiple myeloma.

The cause of the corruption of the plasma cells is unknown, but one possible cause is bombardment by x-rays that can create mutations in the structure of genes, as previously discussed. Another cause may be indicated by the fact that the disease mostly attacks older people. I was 88 when it first occurred; suggesting that an age-related genome mutation may be a factor.

Bone Marrow Biopsy:

Permit me to describe my bone marrow biopsy, because I found it an unnerving experience. I had never had a previous one, and I have now had three. Naive me; I thought the procedure was done by a doctor in surgery rather than by a nurse practitioner in the Infusion Center or on a hospital bed using only a local numbing shot.

I was ushered into a small room with a bed and received a brief description by the nurse practitioner of what was about to happen. I lie face down with my head in a pillow and received the numbing shot above my butt on the right hip bone. The nurse practitioner then began attempts to pierce through the outer layer of the bone into the interior marrow using a sharp instrument similar to what must be similar to an ice pick (I never saw the instrument). I heard the nurse struggling on my backside for several minutes in the attempt to break through to the bone interior. Once she accomplished this, her procedure was to insert a needle through the hole and obtain the marrow material needed. After several more minutes, the nurse announced that the attempt was not successful; she was unable to obtain the material needed since there did not seem to be any fluid in the marrow of my hipbone, so she was terminating the procedure. I was helped to my feet and left the Infusion Center.

Since a bone marrow biopsy is necessary to make a diagnosis, I was scheduled back a week later for another try. It was the same procedure but this time was done on the left hip bone. Again the nurse practitioner struggled for at least five minutes on my back side as I lay face down with my head in a pillow. Finally she announced to an attending nurse that she obtained the fragments she needed but could not obtain any marrow fluid. She excused herself, stepped outside the room and made a phone call to the doctor. Returning, she said the doctor told her he had to have the marrow fluid in order to make a diagnosis – so try again.

At this point, I was turned over to lie on my back so a bone marrow biopsy could be made on my front breast bone. It was the same procedure but this time it was done on my chest in front of my chin – an unnerving experience. After more huffing and puffing and a needle insertion through the hole created in the breast bone, she announced success. She had obtained the marrow liquid. Again, I was helped to my feet and staggered out of the Infusion Center, having survived three bone biopsies. After the numbing shot wore off, intense pain began at the breast site and I was on prescribed pain medication for the following week. The experience added the bone biopsy expertise to my medical resume and it gave me a surgical story to share with other old folks when they started to tell me about their own surgeries.

Treatment:

Multiple myeloma is considered treatable but generally incurable. The principle means of treatment are the utilization of various prescription medications, which include lenalidomide (Revlimid), steroids, chemotherapy, and stem cell transplant (for patients under 65 years of age). Remissions are possible, but rare.

Medications:

In addition to all the other medications I take for my various conditions, which include dermatomyositis, hypertension, high cholesterol, type two diabetes, and gout, I take additional prescriptions for multiple myeloma that include Revlimid, Dexamethasone, and Zometa.

Revlimid (lenalidomide) is a treatment for multiple myeloma. It has significantly improved overall survival in myeloma (which formerly carried a poor prognosis), although toxicity remains an issue for users. [44] The following notes are from the information packet I receive with my prescription:

> "(1): it targets and kills myeloma cells), (2): it helps
> the immune system recognize and destroy myeloma
> cells, and (3): prevents new myeloma cell growth by
> starving them of blood." [45]

Revlimid's exact mechanism of action on cancer cells described on their website is not clear to me. It may be by inhibiting the

---

[44] Revlimid@com, official website, 2017

[45] Revlimid, "Prescription Information, 2017.

growth of new blood vessels in tumors (angiogenesis), enhancing the status of the immune system (through apoptosis –programmed cell death), decreasing cytokine (immo-modulating agents), and growth factor production. [46] I assume all these possibilities are crystal clear to you, even if not to me. (They sound like a script for Tom Cruise from a *Mission Impossible* movie.)

On June 2006, Revlimid received U.S. Food and Drug Administration (FDA) clearance for use in combination with dexamethasone in patients with multiple myeloma who have received at least one prior therapy. On June 2013, the FDA designated Revlimid as a drug requiring a specialty pharmacy distribution. It is only available through a specialty pharmacy's "restricted distribution program in conjunction with a risk evaluation and mitigation strategy." It costs $163,381 per year for the average patient. With the assistance of Dr. Iberri at Stanford Medicine, I received pre-approval of insurance coverage for Revlimid, but even with insurance coverage the co-pay cost is significant and my first year cost for the medication is $10,000.00. [47]

Revlimid is a more potent molecular analog of thalidomide. It is effective at inducing a complete or "very good partial" response as well as improving progression-free survival. Averse events more common in people receiving Revlimid were neutropenia (a decrease in the white blood cell count), deep vein thrombosis, infections, and

---

[46] ibid

[47] "Lenalidomide", Wikimedia, 2017

an increased risk of other malignancies. "The risk does not outweigh the benefit of using Revlimid in multiple myeloma." [48]

The Revlimid protocol is to take one capsule for 21 days, then 7 days of "vacation" with none. (As far as vacations are concerned, I would prefer Miami Beach.)

Dexamethasone is a type of corticosteroid medication. It is used as a direct chemotherapeutic agent in multiple myeloma, in which it is taken in combination with Revlimid. My protocol is to ingest 5 tabs all at the same time on days 1, 8, and 15 of my 21 day Revlimid protocol cycle, with none during the other 7 vacation days. [49] Since it contains a steroid, it also seems to give me a temporary boost.

Zometa (zoledronic acid) was approved by the FDA in 2009 and is administered as an IV and used to prevent skeletal fractures in patients with cancers such as multiple myeloma. It slows down bone resorption (weakening), which is a side effect of multiple myeloma and I am given Zometa as an IV treatment on a monthly basis. [50]

Free light chains: free light chains are a term I have not encountered before and do not fully understand; so, beware

---

[48] ibid

[49] "Revlimid", op, cit.

[50] "Zometa", Wikimedia, 2017

that my description may not be adequate. I am not alone. Their description in the medical literature is vague and confusing.

Free light chains are particle remnants from the corrupted protein molecules in the marrow. They are small subunits of an antibody (immunoglobulin). As I mentioned before, the proteins in the marrow are large organic molecules made even longer with chemical tails (chains) of the molecule that are linked end-to-end. When the molecules become corrupted by multiple myeloma, the long tails become fragmented independent particles that are identified as free light chains and pass through the vascular passageway and into the blood stream. Similar to other protein particles in the blood, free light chains can cause problems. [51]

There are two types of free light chains: *kappa (κ) chain* (its control is located on chromosome 2*)*, and the *lambda (λ) chain* (its control is located on chromosome 22*)*; hence, free light chains are a gene issue. They are kappa or lambda and inherited as the result of a person's genome.

A person's blood contains only one class of free light chain and possesses either kappa or lambda, depending on their genome. For reasons best understood by organic chemical experts, the total kappa to lambda ratio is roughly 3:1. This normal ratio becomes an important number when attempting to count and monitor the quantity of free light chains in a patient's blood. A change

---

[51] "Free Light Chains", Wikipedia, 2017

in the ratio between the two may indicate a metric change in measurement, either good or bad.

Only about one in five people with multiple myeloma produce the free light chain particles that pass into the blood stream. My blood contains the lambda free light chain. Patients with lambda light chain diseases have (reportedly) a three times worse prognosis than those with kappa light chain according to the NIH (National Institute of Health) website, a controversial and questionable conclusion. (Oops, my gene pool may have given me the bad luck of the draw.) [52]

Measurement of free light chains became practical as a clinical blood test in recent years and these tests are used as an aid in the monitoring of multiple myeloma. [53]

Test Results

I receive the results of various blood tests and attempt to monitor the results of my treatment. My knowledge of what the test results actually indicate may be faulty but they do give me motivation to participate in my treatment. Taking twenty pills a day plus all the other sacrifices in my physical wellbeing and lifestyle come with penalties; so, a little motivational boost can go a long way in providing a ray of hope.

---

[52] NIH.GOV, / PMC 2931142

[53] "Free light Chains", Wikipedia, 2017

Here are a few key test results from the past year during the time when I was first diagnosed with multiple myeloma:

	December 2016	March 2017	April 2017	June 2017	August 2017	Sept 2017
Hemoglobin	9.7	10.2	13	13	12.3	12.3

Normal range: (14.0-18.0)

(So my red blood count and hemoglobin remain slightly below the acceptable range)

Lambda Light Chain	87.3	25.31	5.7	4.1	2.8

Normal range: (0.6 – 2.6)

Kappa/Lambda Ratio	<0.1	0.1	0.1	0.3	0.5

Normal range: (0.3 – 1.6)

The numbers of Lambda Light chains found in my blood tests or the results of Kappa/Lambda Ratio are not yet within the acceptable range; however, both of these important results are moving in the correct direction.

My Stanford Specialist:

Please permit me to provide the resume from the internet of Dr. David Iberri who is my specialist and a top practitioner for the treatment of multiple myeloma in the Hematology Department of the Stanford Medical Center. He is a medical oncologist and hematologist who specialize in the treatment of hematologic malignancies. His clinical practice runs the gamut of malignant and non-malignant hematologic disorders including acute and chronic leukemia, multiple myeloma and lymphomas, and bleeding and thrombotic disorders. He is actively involved in clinical trials evaluating novel agents in hematologic malignancies. His research interests are in the development and application of biomarkers to select patients most likely to benefit from therapy.

Academic Appointment:

Clinical Assistant Professor Medicine - Hematology.

Administrative Appointment:

Member, Stanford Professional Evaluation Committee.

Professional Education:

Board Certification: Hematology, American Board of Internal Medicine.

Fellowship: Stanford University School of Medicine (2015)

Board Certification: Internal Medicine, American Board of Internal Medicine.

Residency: Stanford University School of Medicine (2013).

Medical Education: University of Vermont College of Medicine.

I am fortunate to have an excellent specialist such as Dr. Iberri available to guide and assist me with treatment of multiple myeloma.

IN CONCLUSION

There is no end game to multiple myeloma at my age except suffering to be followed by death. Why struggle? Here are some reasons:

I want to experience more of life's events.

To care for my wife and our promise: "until death do us part."

I want to experience more of family – my greatest happiness's are family.

I know I can go above the pain of the final times to focus on family.

www.ingramcontent.com/pod-product-compliance
Lightning Source LLC
Chambersburg PA
CBHW050409290526
45786CB00003B/1190